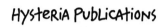

MARIE EVANS &
ANN SHAKESHAFT

THE NOISY PASSAGE

BABY BOOMERS DO MENOPAUSE

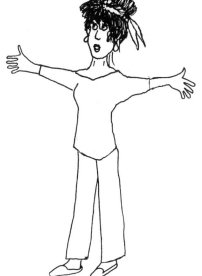

Copyright © 1996 Hysteria Publications
All rights reserved. This book and its parts may not be reproduced in any
form without written permission from the publisher.

Published in the United States by
Hysteria Publications
PO Box 8581
Bridgeport, Connecticut 06605

Deborah Werksman, Publisher
Lysbeth Guillorn, Editor
Nicole Ferentz, Graphic Design
Nancy Moore Brochin, Proofreading and Copy Editing
Tracey Rembert, Internet Research and Word Processing
Barbara Kelly, Sales and Marketing

Cover and interior cartoons by Nicole Hollander

Printed in the United States

ISBN 1-887166-09-2

The information presented herein is for
entertainment only and does not represent medical
advice. It is recommended that readers seek
competent medical attention from a licensed
professional for any matters of personal concern.

MARIE EVANS &
ANN SHAKESHAFT

THE NOISY PASSAGE
BABY BOOMERS DO MENOPAUSE

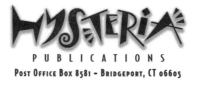

PUBLICATIONS
POST OFFICE BOX 8581 - BRIDGEPORT, CT 06605

Acknowledgments

This book has been written without consent or contribution from any health professionals. Any resemblance to advice received from your gynecologist, acupuncturist, florist, or dentist is strictly coincidental. We especially thank an amateur manicurist, a part-time typist, a passing female cyclist, two Carmelite nuns, and a cocktail waitress for openly sharing their passages with us. We also appreciate the counsel of our doctors, who never returned phone calls. We thank our wonderful children for always hogging the computer and for telling the sixth grade all about menopause.

To our mothers,
who lied and said they
"breezed through it all."

Contents

INTRODUCTION 12

THE NOISY PASSAGE 14
Look Who's Pausin' Now
Your Pausin' Potential
Styles of Pausin': The Name Game

THE EMOTIONAL
ROLLER COASTER 20
Excerpts from the Edge
The Moody Blues
The Pits
Ladies Sing the Blues
A Question of Balance
How to Cure the Blues

HOT FLASH 30
Great Balls of Fire
Red Hot Mamas
Thunder, Lightnin', and Hot Flashes
Where Hot Flashes Strike
The Pausin' Informal Hot Flash Survey
What Not to Say to a Woman Having Hot Flashes

HOOKED ON HORMONES 38
Women on the Verge
The Great Debate
The Decline and Fall of the Hormone Empire
Meet Dr. Hormonowitz

AU NATUREL 47
The Road Best Traveled
Eat to Defeat
Ask Dr. Krystal Ball

THE OBSTACLE COURSE 53
Insomnia: Tossing and Turning
Incontinence: Don't Make Me Laugh
   From Tampax to Depends
   Out of Control
Osteoporosis: Snap, Crackle and Pop
   Is There A Skeleton in Your Closet?
Migraine: The Ultimate Brainstorm
Lost Libido
   Lost and Found

LIVING LARGE 62
Spread Sheet
How Can I Tell If I'm the Right Weight?
Risk Management
The Coming-of-Age Checklist

MALE CORNER 68
Male Tales
Try a Little Tenderness

PAST PAUSE 71
Milestones in Hormones

FUTURE PAUSE-2001: A HORMONE ODYSSEY 75
Surfing the Hormone Superhighway
The Estrological Chart
   The Hormonoscope

PAUSE & REFLECT 82

GLOSSARY 86

ABOUT THE AUTHORS 90

Introduction

THE NOISY PASSAGE WAS WRITTEN for all the women who went to Woodstock, kept their last names, and almost forgot to have families, and by virtue of their huge numbers, continue to set trends.

"The baby boom, known for every stage of life through which it passes, will characteristically make the best of it, transforming the discomforts of menopause into an 'in' passage, a trend—hell, a megatrend!" say Patricia Auberdene and John Naisbitt in *Megatrends for Women*.

As members of the baby boom generation approach 50 (a number previously considered best for speed limits, not age), it will become fashionable to be 50. As Gloria Steinem puts it in her book, *Turning 50*, "Age shouldn't be newsworthy in itself, but it is one more boundary for women to break. Fifty is now what forty used to be."

First you miss a period, so you buy a pregnancy test. You cry at Hallmark commercials, so you call a shrink. You gain five pounds and you replace the elastic in your jogging suit. Forget about it! Look around. In the next few years, female baby boomers with a dwindling supply of hormones will reach epidemic proportions, as 45 million women begin experiencing this change (that's 78.9 pausers per square mile, or half of all female shoppers at Pic and Pay). We have done our best to treat the issues of mood swings, hot flashes, insomnia, weight gain, confusion, memory loss, loss of libido, incontinence, migraines, osteoporosis, and the great hormone debate with the humor and regard that they each deserve.

What's all this meno-madness about? First, let's establish that menopause refers technically to the date of your last menses. This book deals with peri-menopause, the two- to ten-year period that precedes menopause with innumerable symptoms that alter the daily course of women's lives.

Like childbirth, sex, or a double chin, "pausin'," as we call it, can happen quickly and catch you off guard, or it can last for years like a fixed-rate mortgage. With the shutdown of the reproductive system, women face a dilemma— how to handle many symptoms without enough answers. Whatever is a woman to do?

Pausin' is an area of research in its infancy, and unfortunately there is no consensus on how (or if) it should be treated medically. Everyone agrees, however, that the symptoms of pausin' need to be treated with large doses of humor. We wrote *The Noisy Passage* in hopes that it might make humor the second language for all women. *The Noisy Passage* is the survival guide that will cushion the ride!

The Noisy Passage

BY THE END OF THE MILLENNIUM, pausin'
is predicted to create a heated global crisis.
Pause-o-mania may well be the noisiest craze
since Beatlemania, as flower children and former
radicals of the sixties get ready to take hormones
instead of acid and psychedelic mushrooms.

This pause-pandemonium will undoubtedly
wave good-bye to eighties issues, like in-vitro
fertilization and choosing the right school for
your unborn child, in favor of innovative break-
throughs on the hormone frontier. Concerns
over questions ranging from "Will my mail-
order hormones spoil in the back of that hot
UPS truck?" to "What if I fall off the table while
having my Early Bone Density Test?" will make
the Million-Woman March on Washington
the noisiest one yet.

Since there are no absolute answers for
how to deal with the "noisy passage" as of yet,
this book may be the best source to date for
lifting sagging spirits (without surgery).

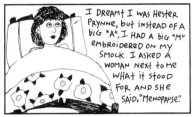 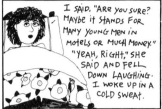

LOOK WHO'S PAUSIN' NOW

In the past, the pausin' milestone was likely to bring out a midlife crisis: women drafted wills, insured their lives, and bought cases of prune juice. But in the nineties, as we sit back and watch science work to reverse the biological clock, no one will be surprised when Calvin, Giorgio, and Yves ask Cindy, Claudia, and Naomi to turn over the runway to their more mature super-sisters!

Let's look at the current "ready-to-pause" crowd: Liza Minelli, Cher, Candace Bergen, Sally Field, Diane Keaton, Susan Sarandon, Naomi Judd, Dolly Parton, Linda Ronstadt, Patty Duke, and Tricia Nixon Cox. And let's not forget about Suzanne (Buns of Steel) Somers, Connie Chung, Charlie's Angels, the Mouseketeers, the Ronnettes, Priscilla Presley, Meryl Streep, Cheryl Tiegs, Olivia Newton-John, Bette Midler, Diane Sawyer, Diana Ross, most Dianes you know, Hilary, Twiggy, Whoopi, Goldie, Ivana, and you! As estro-boomers glide toward 50, we're looking for creative new ways to make pausin' more glamorous (and humorous) as we begin to experience some physical and emotional changes.

Each of us will experience the noisy passage in a different way. Don't be misled by the apparent mystery that surrounds pausin': try to separate the *fact* from the *friction*.

For the most part, the symptoms associated with pausin' are not in themselves a danger to you (only to those around you.

YOUR PAUSIN' POTENTIAL

Some women claim to be symptom-free, even though the age of pause is well upon them. No hot flashes, no irritability, and a good night's sleep! Could this be pausin'? Or is it denial? A small number of women ease into pausin' so gently they don't even know it has come. Most, however, are *more* than aware, and so is everyone around them.

Think you might be pausin'? Find out for sure by taking this harmless twenty-question "Disaster Predictor." The test will measure your hormone level with greater precision than a costly visit to the doctor's office or a blood test with a risky needle.

---

1) Have you recently maimed, dismembered,
   or bludgeoned your secretary, a soccer coach,
   hairdresser, taxi driver, or someone in
   a religious order?   15 points
   Were you arrested and convicted?   3 points
   Did you get away with it?   10 points

---

2) Have you ever filed for divorce or fantasized
   about putting your children up for adoption?   12 points
   Did the divorce come first?   3 points

---

3) Have you decided to have another child
   and discovered that you are a candidate
   for a fertility clinic?   12 points

---

4) Have hot flashes and other discomforts caused you to be demoted or fired as a result of thermostat tampering? 10 points

5) Have you given yourself a frosted home perm or an asymmetrical haircut? 10 points

6) Is your dishwasher spotting, but you're not? 8 points

7) Have you felt under the weather for months due to pre-menstrual, during-menstrual, and after-menstrual syndrome? 8 points

8) Have you misplaced your libido along with your glasses? 8 points

9) Have you been experiencing jet-lag without leaving your home? 8 points

10) Have you experienced the "aura" associated with hot flashes, but not seen Elvis? 8 points

11) Have "one size fits all" labels crept into your closet? 7 points

12) Have you had a minor brush with the law for a rush-hour traffic violation? 7 points

13) Are you having unexplainable crying spells, even though you have just been given a raise and a promotion? 6 points

14) Have your hips and thighs gotten heavier as your periods have gotten lighter? 6 points

15) Are your mood swings setting the pace for office parties? 6 points

16) Have constant bouts of anxiety and depression made it impossible to concentrate on your bank balance? 5 points

17) Is R-E-M being disturbed at night by P-E-E?	3 points

18) Have the headaches you lied about for so many years finally surfaced as the real thing?	1 point

19) Do you still believe that cosmetics can help your skin?	-5 points

20) Has anyone used the word "hot" in the same sentence as your name in the last two years? (doctors don't count)	-5 points
In the last two weeks?	-10 points

Your Total:

EVALUATION:

The higher your total score, the lower your estrogen level.

If you received this many points...	You are probably...
0-5	Still in college
6-30	Still in denial
31-45	On the cusp
45-60	In full swing

STYLES OF PAUSIN'

The Name Game

As we no longer live in a world where one stylistic viewpoint predominates, pausin', like decorating, reflects a wide range of styles and attitudes. Diversity of expression is the hallmark of the modern woman. Which category best suits your pausin' style? Use the chart below and compare the name with the pause-style. Draw a line between each style and each personality.

Style	Personality
Modern	Betsey Johnson
Victorian	Paloma Picasso
Country	Marilyn Quayle
Hi-Tech	Annie Lennox
Art Deco	Dolly Parton
Colonial	Bernadette Peters
Louis XVI	Anne Rice
Traditional	Camille Paglia
Eclectic	Princess Anne

The Emotional Roller Coaster

DO YOU FEEL OUT OF CONTROL? Is the Screamin' Demon a ride at Great Escape or your nickname? Formerly known as nervous breakdowns, mood swings can seem a capricious romp, a psychotic rave or merely a confrontation with your Inner Bitch. At least half of all peri-menopausal American women experience mood swings. Yours may be precipitated by "routine" domestic developments, such as your son losing your car, or your daughter and you both discovering you are pregnant at the same time. Mood swings are responsible for the large numbers of women of a certain age behind bars (both prisons and pubs).

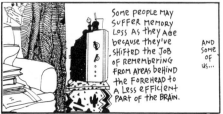
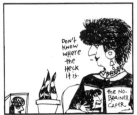

EXCERPTS FROM THE EDGE

"My crying at the dinner table has upset my husband and children, but I really feel refreshed when I'm done and it adds to my food the extra salt I've been craving." —Jane, head chef at an Upper East Side bistro

"Eye to eye with the prison gynecologist, I found myself breathlessly repeating that old refrain, 'Make my day.'"
—Patty, serving five years for carrying a concealed weapon

"I was crying all the time. Then I found Bailey's Irish Creme. Now I keep a bottle in my desk drawer. AA has been really helpful and I've made a lot of new friends." —Betty, CEO at a major pharmaceutical company

"Mood swings would sneak up on me in the middle of the night. I hope I didn't wake my neighbors when I started the jackhammer." —Susan, performance artist

THE MOODY BLUES

Raging hormonal turbulence invades a woman's life three times:

1st: During the teen years: The figure starts to round out and swell, giving it a softer and more sensual look. This produces tantrums, inappropriate behavior, relentless confrontations with mothers (minipause meets menopause) and an inexplicable attraction to boys. This is the first stage of PMS.

2nd: During pregnancy: The swell balloons into exorbitant abundance. This produces whining, weeping, and hemorrhoids. Double the PMS.

3rd: Pausin': The abundance continues to abound. This, added to all of the previously mentioned symptoms (with the exception of boys), produces courage, unusual solutions to everyday problems, and an irresistible desire to run for public office.

THE PITS

Anxiety, Depression, Fatigue and Irritability are the four most popular destinations of women traveling on the "Hormone Superhighway." Typically, before other signs of pausin' emerge, such as skipping a period or feeling the need to adopt a child, the pausin' woman starts to feel like a frayed nerve ending with legs.

Anxiety: You wake in the middle of the night and obsess about the deterioration of the ozone layer.

Depression: You can't return phone calls because if anyone is nice to you, you'll start to cry.

Fatigue: You hate yourself and everybody else in the morning. You sleep till noon, but you're still too tired to call the therapist.

Irritability: You see ineptitude everywhere, there are no good shows on TV, and you're out of vodka.

The phenomenon of pausin' leaves many women (and doctors) bewildered and confused. As a woman's behavior runs from mild to wild, she may be struggling to maintain hormonal harmony and make sense of what is happening to her mind and body. By following the diagnostic road map on the next pages, you can find out which symptoms have the most impact on your feelings.

ANXIETY:

- Have chapped lips kept you from wearing your favorite shades of lipstick?
- Have you abused chemical peels to the point of hospitalization?
- Have you been forbidden to engage in hobbies like needlepoint because a sharp object is involved?
- Is it more satisfying to work out at the rifle range than at the gym?
- Do you suffer from "pink-eye" as a result of seeing red all the time?
- Do you feel anxious most of the time or just when going for oral surgery?
- Have you recently given up your favorite talk show or cigarettes?
- Have you been considering buying a new bathing suit?

DIAGNOSIS:

Feelings of tension, apprehension, and edginess, accompanied by palpitations or excessive shopping sprees are normal during pausin'. If you answered "Yes" to two or more of the above questions, however, your anxiety may stem from phobias about your computer losing its memory or chipping a nail. Stop gnawing at your nails and resume alcohol, cigarettes, and chocolate at once.

DEPRESSION:

- Are Happy Meals no longer doing the job?
- Has the onset of depression followed a distressing event, such as your ice-maker breaking down?

- Are you pregnant?
- Are you over 60?
- Are you over 60 and pregnant?
- Have you recently experienced multiple births resulting from fertility drug abuse? *(If so, see "Nannies" in the Yellow Pages.)*
- Have you accidentally mixed hormones with tanning gel or hemorrhoid cream?
- Are you taking more pills now than you did in college and high school?
- Have you recently had to give up hormone replacement therapies and alcohol at the same time?
- Are daily chocolate binges giving you diarrhea? *(If so, investigate chocolate substitutes such as pecan pie and banana splits.)*
- Have you recently discovered that even the Wonder Bra doesn't help?

DIAGNOSIS:

Answering "YES" to even one of these questions means you may be suffering from feelings of sadness, futility, and despair that make it impossible for you to cope with normal life situations such as stray dogs, untamed children, demanding bosses, and unmanageable hair. These feelings are perfectly normal during pausin', but be careful not to confuse depression with routine household chores.

FATIGUE:

- When you make your bed, do you only think about getting back in it?
- Do you do the dishes sitting down?
- Do you feel a sense of accomplishment by walking from the bed to the fridge?

- Have you collected more take-out menus than cobwebs in your house?
- Does watching exercise videos make you tired?
- Have you fired your personal fitness trainer or let your gym membership lapse?
- Have you considered signing up for Meals on Wheels, but are too tired to fill out the application?
- Do you continue to cancel doctors' appointments even thought you are running out of pills?

DIAGNOSIS:

It is safe to assume that most women will answer "Yes" to all of the above questions. Exhaustion has become a way of life for most women. Juggling home, job, children, and doctors' appointments is enough to sap any woman's energy. Recently, heightened energy surges were reported when hormone replacement therapy was taken in conjunction with six-packs of Jolt cola and when someone found a pastry chef willing to make housecalls.

IRRITABILITY:

- When you enter the room do people stop talking and leave quietly?
- Does the dog leave too?
- Have you repeated simple directions to your employees, children or mate more than 3 times in 15 minutes, i.e., "Get me the Tums, get me the Tums, get me the Tums"?
- Has your tone of voice taken on a strident edge or are you experiencing a tightness and clicking in your jaw due to permanent wrath?
- Is a single glass of wine no longer able to soothe your nerves?
- A full bottle?

- Do you feel out of control over silly things like upper arm flab?
- Are you guilty of aggressive acts towards complete strangers?

DIAGNOSIS:

The edginess and impatience of irritability are often misunderstood as nagging. Irritability is no laughing matter, and flagrant displays of it will usually get you off jury duty. We recommend pot smoking, love-ins, and sitar music as vehicles to help you regain your tranquility, combined with political activism, late night dancing, and strenuous sports to help you vent your spleen.

LADIES SING THE BLUES

High levels of progesterone or a drop in estrogen levels are responsible for the erratic mood swings that plague women during the pausin' years and, as chance would have it, the topic of every book written by a president's wife.

STRESS MANAGEMENT

The panel on Panic Prevention for Mid-life Crisis gives the following tips to control stress and mood swings, good for even the most mild-mannered pauser:

- Remember that all the moms on "Nick at Nite" are fictitious.
- Mood rings are synonymous with medic alert buzzers, so wear yours at all times.
- The fashion industry and royalty are good midlife career changes for women with mood swings; they are considered signs of creativity and superiority.

• Join your local "Swingers" club for additional support (and fun).

A QUESTION OF BALANCE

As a general rule of thumb, hormonally balanced women do not participate in the following activities. Check the box(es) below which apply to your own behavior.

☐ Cry when reading the phone book
☐ Report neighbors for minor sanitation violations
☐ Make prank delivery calls to the local pizza parlor
☐ Drive in demolition derbies
☐ Make paté out of small furry animals
☐ Apply for a gun permit
☐ Call personal psychics more than seven times per week
☐ Send inflatable love dolls to the president
☐ Rip the door off the hinges when the key doesn't fit
☐ Sleep with power tools under the pillow in case the urge to remodel surges
☐ Lick the center out of Oreos and leave the empty cookies for your kids
☐ Make nocturnal visits to the ice-maker
☐ Chase every meal with a pint of Ben & Jerry's ice cream
☐ Shave in public pools

If you checked this many boxes...	You are probably...
0-5	still staying in line
5-10	progressing to borderline
10-15	walking a fine line
15-20	approaching the finish line

28 / The Noisy Passage: Baby Boomers Do Menopause

HOW TO CURE THE BLUES

Once you are "in full swing" of pausin', you may want to consider finding the right doctor. Many of the doctors that women rely on for years question whether hot flashes, PMS, and other symptoms of pausin' really exist or are only excuses to get out of picking up the dry cleaning .

Before you fill your prescriptions, fill in the blanks with the following names—find out just how much you know about selecting Dr. Right.

Dr. Ruth	Dr. Welby	Dr. Zhivago
Dr. Pepper	Dr. Kildare	Doc Gooden
Dr. Doolittle	Dr. Frankenstein	Doc Adams
Dr. Strangelove	Dr. Kevorkian	Dr. Seuss
Dr. Spock		

1) For loss of libido, I would call _____ .

2) I feel like a monster inside needs to come out. I think _____ can best help me.

3) _____ will know how to pitch me a good exercise regimen and workout!

4) To quench my thirst after a hot flash, I always turn to _____ .

5) For a good movie to cool me down, I'd call _____ .

6) If I'm feeling depressed and need to be cheered, _____ is who I'd see.

7) When I find myself having long, meaningful dialogues with my pet ferret, I call _____ .

8) _____ can end all my troubles
   when I've had enough and just can't take it anymore.

9) For fractures, broken bones, and limping,
   I'd call _____ .

10) I could revitalize my energy for a romp with
    _____ .

11) To defuse my atomic hot flashes,
    _____ is the one I need.

12) To set the record straight about pausin',
    _____ has all the answers.

13) When my Inner Bitch needs to get in touch with
    my Inner Child, I read _____ .

Hot Flash

HOT FLASH IS TO PAUSIN' what nacho is to chips, what cellulite is to thighs and what Beavis is to Butthead. Hot flashes are becoming so prevalent due to the large number of pausers, that they could put fans, freon, and Eskimo Pies on a list of hot stocks to consider. Like Godzilla approaching Tokyo, this molten monster attacks unsuspecting women, ruthlessly bringing on soaring temperatures, spontaneous combustion, and third-degree burns. First there's a spark, then there's dynamite. Like a bolt out of the blue, a hot flash hits your head and comes out of your shoe.

Not to worry. Women struck by hot flashes have a 99% survival rate, with a 100% survival rate for those who regularly change the batteries in their smoke detectors. Women today see hot flashes as tremendous power surges that can open nasal passages and bottles of Dom Perignon as quickly as they can open doors to new careers.

GREAT BALLS OF FIRE

"When I experience a flash at work I walk quickly to the ladies room, remove my jacket and blouse, and press myself up against the cool tiles until the feeling subsides. A quick touch-up in the mirror and I'm as good as new." —Marge, ticket clerk in Grand Central Terminal

"I have taken to stripping down to my unmentionables during the day while doing household chores. I know that this has been a topic of conversation for the U.P.S. men in our region, but I am much more comfortable. Plus, delivery service has been excellent!"
—Alana, homemaker and skin care consultant

"Imagine my embarrassment when I experienced a hot flash at my daughter's high school car wash. I pretended to forget to roll up my car window so I could get a quick hosedown. (It felt great!)"
—Hilary, P.T.A. president

"A hot flash is a natural resource with a mighty powerful potential." —Bonnie, PR directory, public utility

"I woke up drenched in a pool of perspiration. It was so refreshing, I started to do the backstroke."
—Donna, former Olympic bronze medalist in swimming

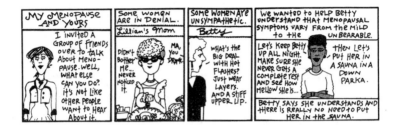

RED HOT MAMAS

For centuries, women have pondered how to control hot flashes. In ancient times, hot flashes were looked upon as powerful and deadly weapons, belonging only to the gods. Today, by tracing this "soggy symptom" through the pages of history, we find that hot flashes are not simply a fictitious "flash in the pan," but actual, celebrated historic events.

WHY WAS:

- Shiva engulfed in flames?
- Botticelli's Venus sailing on a clam shell?
- Marilyn Monroe standing over a breezy subway grate?
- The Statue of Liberty standing in the middle of New York Harbor wearing only a toga?
- Duchamp's nude descending the staircase?
- Lady Godiva hot to trot?

Remember that as much as men would like to believe that we spend every waking moment creating new ways to attract their attention, this is not exactly true. Like Pavlov's dogs, men can often be found sniffing around a hot flash, hoping that flimsier clothing choices will result in a meeting of the minds (at the very least). Down, boys!

THUNDER, LIGHTNIN', AND HOT FLASHES

Hot flashes are setting off smoke alarms across the country to the scale of a pyrotechnic extravaganza. Scientists predict that as millions of women throughout the world simultaneously experience them, temperatures will soar and accelerate the greenhouse effect. Here are some of the most often asked questions about hot flashes:

Q: Am I safe in a bathtub during a hot flash?
A: The bathtub is the safest place through all your pausin' years. Pruny skin is a small price to pay for your dignity. Limit soaking time if you notice peeling wallpaper.

Q: If I am outdoors, where should I seek shelter from a hot flash?
A: Keep a low profile when having a hot flash out in a field. Burrowing yourself into a hole is a good idea if you don't mind messing up a French manicure.

Q: Is it dangerous to have a hot flash in an airplane?
A: Yes, because the bathroom sink is usually too small to accommodate an adult body.

Q: Is it true that a hot flash never strikes twice?
A: No. Hot flashes often hit the "biggest" thing around. Which means the Sears Tower in Chicago, the Empire State Building in New York, or you!

Q: Should you disconnect your appliances during a hot flash?
A: It is not necessary to disconnect them as long as you don't overtax the circuit breaker by using too many appliances at once. Appliance abuse (fans, refrigerators, ice makers, exercise machines, frozen drink makers...) is an overlooked symptom of pausin'.

Q: Is it true that rubber-soled shoes are the best choice for someone who is experiencing hot flashes?
A: Yes, rubber shoes or boots will hold the sweaty runoff from a hot flash until you have the opportunity to empty them, thus covering your tracks, so to speak.

Q: Is it safe to talk on the phone during a hot flash?
A: Many women have no trouble doing two or even more things at the same time, like cooking, talking on the phone, and keeping their children out of the washing machine.

WHERE HOT FLASHES STRIKE

Hot flashes occur when diminished levels of estrogen irritate certain neuroreceptors in the base of the brain. These neuroreceptors in turn signal the blood vessels to expand, the blood vessels then heat up the skin and *voilà*—fireworks! Many women describe this as a feeling of warmth passing over the body as if it were being draped in a plush sable coat. Others reported a drenching sweat followed by chills. Statistics show that 85% of women will experience hot flashes. That's more than will experience finding a place for holiday leftovers in the refrigerator.

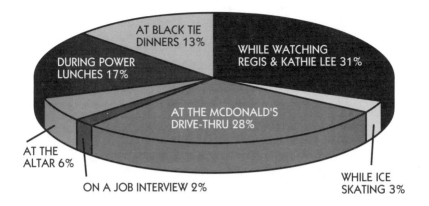

THE PAUSIN' INFORMAL HOT FLASH SURVEY

How would you describe your hot flashes?

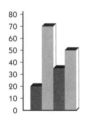

1) Spontaneous and Sassy!
   "Bring 'em on, I can handle it"
2) Slam, Bam, Thank You Ma'am
   "Like a knockout punch"
3) Slow Boil
   "Yes, yes, don't stop"
4) Earth-Shaking
   "I'm on fire"

What will you change next time?

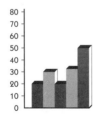

1) Wouldn't change a thing
2) Underwear
3) I'd wear dress shields
4) The sheets
5) My attitude

Where would you prefer to have a hot flash?

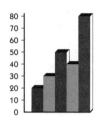

1) In bed
2) The shower
3) In a bathing suit
4) After a romantic dinner
5) In another life

Which of these things can invigorate your interest in a hot flash?

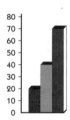

1) Videos on Antarctica
2) A Cool Whip massage
3) Snowmen

Have you ever experienced loss of interest in hot flashes?

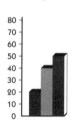

1) Yes, during the flu season
2) When given the cold shoulder
3) I have pledged to remain flash-free until I am married

WHAT NOT TO SAY TO A WOMAN HAVING HOT FLASHES

This is a sensitive time for pausers. One wrong word and your life could be on the line. Here are some remarks to avoid:

- "Are your pantyhose cutting off your circulation?"
- "It's women like you who are melting the polar ice caps."
- "With a gal like you, I can save on heating bills."
- "You're *still* having hot flashes?"
- "Does this mean you are going to give up on trying to have a baby?"
- "I think I'd be more comfortable in single beds."
- "You've got a little mascara under your eye."
- "I forgot to refill the ice cube tray."
- "Is there a wet t-shirt contest going on?"
- "Did you just come from the gym?"
- "They were sold out of convertibles."
- "I bought you a wet suit for your birthday."
- "You look great, wet or dry."
- "Would you mind standing a little closer? There are a few wrinkles left in my suit."

Hooked on Hormones

ARE YOU WITHDRAWING FROM HORMONES LIKE a junkie going cold turkey? Would you welcome a little relief? At first, many women choose to treat their symptoms with the least invasive means—chicken soup with a little garlic— while others (previously tolerant of opiates and hallucinogens) go straight for the drugs!

But hormones aren't a panacea. Plus, finding the right dose, whether it be in the form of a patch, a pill, or a papaya, can be an arduous process, rivaled only by finding a Xerox machine in your office that won't break down after being repeatedly punched, kicked and maligned.

Since gynecologists pass out hormones like M&M's, estrogen has become the #1 prescribed drug in America. Some swear it's the closest thing to an elixir of youth that modern medicine has to offer, while others complain of the side effects.

In the final analysis, you may be better off with a good psychoanalyst.

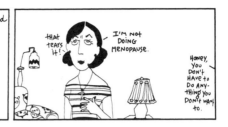

WOMEN ON THE VERGE

"I had been getting mean and edgy, but didn't realize that my behavior could be traced to hormone impairment. Well, the sad truth is, before I could get the help I needed, I bludgeoned my husband to death when he refused to give me the TV remote control."

—Dee Dee, doing life with no parole (and no TV privileges)

"I wanted to pick up the refrigerator and throw it out the window. My rage was simply unexplainable. It was worse than a bad acid trip."

—Dot, psychiatric clinic outpatient

"My husband has been so understanding of my mood swings. He offers to cook dinner for us and then gives me a relaxing massage. As a reward, I split my estrogen with him; it makes him feel better to know that we are going through this together." —Laurie, divorce attorney

"I used to be even-tempered, then I started to have psychotic experiences. I found it impossible to be around my 11 children. I started low doses of estrogen and now things have changed so much that I even adopted a few dogs. My favorite is the Golden Retriever; he understands me and you should see how sweetly he licks my face when I have a hot flash."

—Turquoise, resident of Rainbow Hills ashram

THE GREAT DEBATE

Hormone Replacement Therapy (HRT) has been surrounded by so much controversy that many women have difficulty charting the best course through the minefield of menopause. Who should take HRT? How much should be taken? How little? When to start? When to stop? These questions can put a damper on your already damp life.

Basically the message today regarding HRT is that hormones increase your chances of getting breast cancer at 60, while helping prevent a hip fracture at age 70. If by chance you are considering HRT, the chart on the following page may help you see the pros and cons of hormone consumption.

With HRT	Without HRT
strong nails	campaign trails
bouncy and glossy hair	bouncy personality
awesome sex	turbo metabolism
memory rejuvenation	period cessation
breast enlargement	clean mammogram
the comfort of chills	no pills, no bills
smooth, glowing complexion	no worries about conception
ample, bee-stung lips	shapely legs and hips
uplifted butt	spirited strut
carefree days	no drug haze
perpetual lubrication	good Pap smear
brightened outlook	Oprah's cookbook

THE DECLINE AND FALL
OF THE HORMONE EMPIRE

For a few women, hormones can be almost 100% effective in relieving hot flashes, mood swings, and traffic violations. However, taking hormones can involve some health risks and some side effects.

So, if you are experiencing irregular cycles, and a bad temper, and find that chocolate no longer does the job, you may turn to something stronger. Each of us needs to find a personal solution to our distinctive set of problems. Listed below are some of the most popular methods to treat pausin' with and without tricks. See also the section on natural remedies.

BIRTH CONTROL PILLS

Birth control pills are often the first replacement therapy prescribed. This is excellent, because even women who don't have mood swings react badly to becoming pregnant when they are in the twilight of their forties.

ESTROGEN

Estrogen, the female hormone, comes in a variety of forms, but not flavors. Patches are the newest form of estrogen replacement. When worn together with patches designed for nicotine and motion sickness, you will be able to accompany anyone, anywhere, anytime! Patches come in small, medium, and large, and coordinate with your dress size (X-large can be custom made). Estrogen pills are commonly used and taken daily. However, on special occasions, like high school reunions, wedding anniversaries, and tennis tournaments, you may want to splurge.

SUPPOSITORIES AND CREAMS

Vaginal inserts increase lubrication, and supply all the estrogen needed. Overzealous users even attest to remarkable skin improvements, including the disappearance of liver spots and adult acne. The main drawback of estrogen cream is that it is messy—especially when standing up.

PROGESTERONE

Progesterone, like estrogen, comes in several synthetic forms. Progesterone is said to protect the uterus, and is well worth taking if you can bear the side effects of fatigue, water retention, swollen and tender breasts, vaginal dryness, and loss of libido, all in tandem with erratic mood swings. Coincidentally, this is the #1 reason women stop taking HRT, resume alcohol, and become celibate.

TESTOSTERONE

Testosterone is a male hormone included in some HRT programs to increase sex drive and response. It is usually administered in pill form. Testosterone has recently been added to the list of controlled substances, because it has certain side effects. Some tell-tale signs of trouble are:

Too Much of a Good Thing

- Widening of the upper arms and torso
- Unusual fascination with guns and computers
- Dramatic improvement in your golf handicap
- The dog becomes your best friend
- Snoring loudest in the family
- Wearing BVDs rather than an IUD
- ESPN takes over QVC
- Determination to change your own tires
- Resisting asking for directions no matter how lost you are
- Deep voice
- Increased libido
- 5 o'clock shadow

Warning: Keep all hormones away from teenagers prone to bodybuilding.

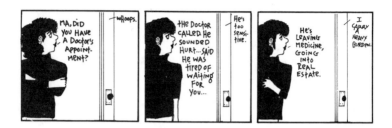

MEET DR. HORMONOWITZ

Meet Dr. Mona Hormonowitz, gynecologist to the stars. Dr. Hormonowitz takes her vow of confidentiality seriously, so she can't name names. Let's just say she's ridden the hormonal roller coaster with Hollywood's finest. Now, by popular demand (and to pay off a hefty malpractice suit), Dr. Hormonowitz has agreed to share her gems of gynecological wisdom with the masses.

Dear Dr. Hormonowitz:
I'm a 42-year-old married mother of two teenagers. I chose birth control pills as my form of HRT because my doctor assured me that they contain just the right blend of estrogen and progesterone for my peri-menopausal needs. Two months ago, during a rare mood swing, my bottle of pills fell out of my pocket when I attempted to climb in off the ledge of my apartment building. Last week my doctor informed me that I can expect to hear the pitter patter of little feet in eight months and two weeks. I assume she is not forecasting the arrival of a companion for our pet schnauzer. Doctor—how did this happen?

—Great with Child

Dear Great:
It is entirely conceivable for a healthy 42-year-old woman to become pregnant. Just look at Murphy Brown. She managed to conceive a child at your age, to give birth to a bouncing baby, and to juggle a successful career and motherhood. Not only that, she was picked up for another season. I'm sure the same will be true for you.

—*MH*

Dear Dr. Hormonowitz:
Until recently I've been using Premarin, the estrogen supplement derived from the urine of pregnant horses. It gave me a dewy soft complexion and brought back my libido. So, when I received the invitation to my 25th high school reunion last spring, I decided to splurge and double my dosage. I figured I'd wow them at the reunion with my youthful good looks. The plan backfired. I developed an insatiable craving for oats, hay, and wide open spaces. I immediately stopped taking the Premarin, but what do I do about the reunion?

—*An Old Gray Mare*

Dear Mare:
The perfect solution to your problem is an estrogen patch, which my dear friend Versace says makes the perfect accessory for that knock-out dress you're planning to wear to your reunion!

—*MH*

Dear Dr. Hormonowitz:
I'm a 51-year-old car salesperson who is rapidly losing her libido. My boyfriend says it's because I'm taking progesterone, which tends to diminish the desire to be fondled, touched, looked at, or breathed upon. Three months ago, he convinced me to start taking testosterone to increase my sex drive. The good news is that not only do I feel like making love all the time, but I can also change a flat tire on the used car lot without using a jack. The bad news is that I have 5 o'clock shadow and my voice has dropped three octaves. What should I do?

—Crazed and Confused

Dear Crazed:
Learn to take the good with the bad. Facial hair and a deep voice made a fortune for Barry White. And Barry would have had to call AAA to change that tire.

—MH

Au Naturel

HOW MANY OF US HAVE SPENT YEARS chasing diaphragms across bathroom floors after being scared off birth control pills, and naturally puffed and breathed our way into motherhood, declining the "saddleblock?" You've put Redi-Whip, beef jerky, Spam, and Velveeta behind you, so why tolerate chemicals in the modern medical form so quickly? Many women have found relief from herbal remedies, and very few have ever experienced unwanted hallucinations.

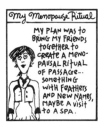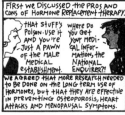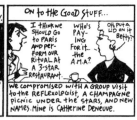

THE ROAD BEST TRAVELED

The natural approach to address the symptoms of pausin' is multi-dimensional. Listed here are some popular remedies used to lessen the symptoms. Some are a bit risky, others are still shaky, and some are downright on the fringes. By placing the words from the list in the appropriate columns, you will be able to measure your home remedy savvy.

Juniper berries	Alcohol	Fluoride
Yams	Birkenstock sandals	Listerine
Yucca	Incense	Nicotine
Aromatherapy	Bubble bath	Oysters
Primal therapy	Buddhism	*People* magazine
Wheat grass	Caffeine	Robitussin
Shark cartilage	Caftans	Special K
Burdock root	Chocolate	Alfalfa sprouts
Yoga	Pickles	Tanning gel
Chromium	Decaf Diet Coke	Tofu
Beta carotene	Evian water	Dong Quai
Herbal tea	Gravy	Acupuncture
Ginseng	Chanel No.5	Power lunch
Fresh vegetables	Prunes	Nuts and berries
Canned heat	Prune danish	Nuts and bolts

Homeopathic	Herbal	Pure Magic	Habit Forming	Mind Blowing

EAT TO DEFEAT

As an alternative to hormone replacement therapy, there's a new list of natural foods that are said to relieve hot flashes, dryness, and mood swings; there's even talk that these same items ward off impotence—so ladies, hide your stash!

Foods such as soy and cruciferous vegetables (broccoli, kale, cabbage, Brussels sprouts, etc.) contain rich sources of "phytoestrogen" (plant hormones), which regulate our hormonal metabolism to a more favorable balance and protect against estrogen-related cancers. Whipped cream, coffee, and nachos are now your enemies; wild yams, chaste tree berries, and filet of mung are now your new friends.

Armed with these facts and the following shopping list, you can now navigate the aisles of your nearest Tofu 'R' Us with an air of knowing superiority.

SHOPPING LIST FOR THE HORMONALLY CHALLENGED

Twinkie extract: The essence of the Twinkie experience without all that sugar and fat.

Shmoffee: A tasty noncaffeinated coffee substitute made from dried carob, sawdust, and burnt cork shavings— for that just-brewed flavor.

Birch bark: Do not eat! For the woman suffering from caffeine withdrawal (see item above), bark strips can be woven into lovely placemats to keep those idle hands busy.

Eau de Lady Who Sweats: Sparkling mineral water for the woman in need of a cold flash.

Can o' Yams: An instant treat to smooth out those violent mood swings. This item boasts user-friendly packaging: any woman can open this with her teeth and eat directly from the can.

Two-day-old whole-grain loaf: Good for sharpening teeth (see item above) and, when aimed properly, an effective weapon against anyone who crosses you.

Ben & Jerry's chocolate chip cookie dough ice cream: Two pints completely demolish any cravings for chocolate chip cookies.

ASK DR. KRYSTAL BALL

Dr. Krystal Ball is a syndicated advice columnist specializing in alternative treatments for pausin'. In 1996 she received her doctorate in Advanced Herbal Psychobotany from the Decaffeinated Mocha Latte Correspondence School in Chokeberry, California. Dr. Ball encourages her readers to write about their problems instead of acting them out. She believes that the pen is mightier than the sword (a pauser herself, she has tried both; she is now on work release from Sunny Side State penitentiary).

Dear Dr. Ball:
I am 49 years old and trying aromatherapy for the first time to balance out the strange mood swings I've been experiencing lately. Last night, I brought home some healing oils, but the smell overpowered my burning macaroni and cheese casserole. Can you give me some tips on distinguishing the smell of slippery elm bark from that of burning food?

—Rebel Without a Clue

Dearest Rebel:
Are you aware that when mixed with cedar fungus and a pinch of milkweed shavings, slippery elm bark makes a tangy side dish for macaroni and cheese? Always remember: When the Goddess closes a door, somewhere she opens a window (which you might try next time for better kitchen ventilation).

—KB

Dear Krystal:
I've been using massage therapy to relieve the anxiety, depression, stress, and occasional homicidal tendencies brought on by menopause. My massage therapist, Fabio, is so talented that I am now able to achieve intense mellowness. I become one not

only with my higher self, but also with the massage table. Here's my conflict: I've become addicted to massage. The only oil I use nowadays is preheated, my office desk has been outfitted with black leather cushions, my wardrobe has been replaced by a sack of white towels, and Fabio recently moved his Barca-Lounger into my den. Please, Krystal, how can I kick the massage habit? My goal is to wean myself to 12 sessions per week.

—*Sleepless in Seattle*

Dear, dear Sleepless:
It is truly a blessing that you and Fabio have gotten in touch with your body. My question to you is, why wean yourself at all? My advice is to build a small wing on the end of your house and invite Fabio to live in. With some training, he could probably also empty the dishwasher and make a great cup of herbal tea. —*KB*

Dear Krys:
My acupuncturist claims that by pressing on certain acu-pressure points on my own body, I can relieve many menopausal symptoms. For instance, she told me that by pressing my left index finger against the bridge of my nose, I can rid myself of migraine headaches. As it turns out, she is correct. But I do want to warn your readers that I experienced a downside to this self-treatment during an auction I attended last month. Sensing the beginnings of a migraine, I pressed my acu-pressure point and am now the owner of an $8,000 Louis XIV carriage clock.   —*No Way Out*

Dear No Way:
Perhaps by meditating on the clock, you can channel Louis IV. Think of this as a wonderful opportunity for time travel.

—*KB*

The Obstacle Course
Insomnia, Incontinence, Migraines, Lost Libido, Osteoporosis

INSOMNIA, INCONTINENCE, AND MIGRAINES aren't always associated with pausin' (especially by doctors), but mark our words, if you are in your 40s and start to notice changes in your "perpendicular performance" or loss of control between your ears and legs, you had better believe it's estrogen driven. Still, howling at the moon, never uncrossing your legs, or feeling like an elephant is standing on your forehead seems inconsequential in comparison to the distress caused by some other symptoms of pause.

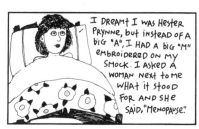 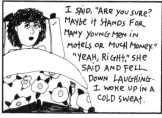

INSOMNIA
Tossing and Turning

Insomnia, like many other symptoms of pausin', occurs as a result of estrogen reduction. Hot flashes, anxiety, nightmares, pins and needles, peri-incontinence, night sweats and forgetting to marinate tomorrow night's dinner are just a few sources of poor nightly performance. This nocturnal restlessness that shaves hours off a pauser's sleep can greatly interfere with a general sense of well-being, but surveys have shown that insomniacs accomplish more than their better-rested peers.

If you are experiencing a burst of energy between 2:00 and 5:00 am, this may be the perfect time to:

• apply to a Ph.D. program

• take up sculpting on a large scale

• run for public office

• write a novel

• create your own brand of perfume

• start up a small business

INCONTINENCE
Don't Make Me Laugh

FROM TAMPAX TO DEPENDS

If you think that losing control of your bladder suggests the deterioration of one more body function, you are correct! For years doctors have espoused the Kegel exercise (squeezing exercises designed to strengthen the muscles that support the bladder and uterus) as an antidote for incontinence... but for many women it's anticlimactic (so to speak).

Don't be caught off guard. Buy a watch with an alarm (at this stage in your life, water-resistant is best). Set the alarm and empty your bladder every hour. This practice will keep you dry, and two steps ahead of disaster. You never know when someone will lean over in the middle of a sales conference and whisper a funny joke in your ear, or when pollen season might cause a sneezing fit.

OUT OF CONTROL

To see how severe your condition is, take this simple true or false test.

	TRUE	FALSE
Your family always complains about the frequent stops when traveling by car.		
You place a nursing pad under the sheets on your side of the bed to protect the mattress.		
You have developed a taste for cranberry juice.		
An autographed 8x10 glossy of June Allyson adorns your bathroom.		
You have given up aerobics for yoga.		
Although you use Tampax only for your sporadic periods, the cabinet below the sink is packed with extra-absorbency sanitary napkins and pads.		

	TRUE	FALSE
Roller coasters and amusement parks are not so amusing anymore.		
You are experiencing the same nocturnal bathroom habits that you had when you were eight months pregnant.		

If you were able to complete this test without going to the bathroom, your bladder is still in good shape. Don't despair. If you went once, there is hope. Try these additional tips to help you curb the urge.

- Always sit in the aisle seat in theaters, and in airplanes and other forms of transportation, assuring you quicker access to the bathroom.

- Avoid comedy clubs.

- Discontinue vitamins—they color your urine, making spotting a laundry nightmare.

- Avoid car travel without updated maps of Interstate rest stops.

- Remember: the bulging outline of even the most streamlined adult diaper is a dead giveaway, so avoid wearing bicycle shorts or that miniskirt from your Woodstock revival party.

If you read this on the toilet, not even this book can help you.

OSTEOPOROSIS
Snap, Crackle & Pop

Many people each year fall and break a hip as a result of osteoporosis. By answering the following questions, you can assess your risk and see if you are a possible candidate for becoming the human equivalent of a box of peanut brittle.

1. Did your mother ever shatter anything other than her dishes?

2. Are you the same height now that you were at 25? (Deduct 8 inches if you wore a beehive)?

3. Do you rate your overall health as poor, very poor, or just plain fed up?

4. Do your teeth and breath scream espresso abuse?

5. Do you spend less than an hour on your feet each day, even when wearing Birkenstocks?

6. Do you rarely walk for exercise unless you are going to the liquor store?

7. Are you unable to rise from a chair without using your arms, the chair's arms, or other people's arms?

8. Is your resting pulse more than 80 beats a minute?

9. Do you think "break dancing" is for the over-the-hill generation?

10. Did you break any bones (spouse's don't count) after age 50?

Answering "yes" to five or more questions means you are 16 times more likely to have osteoporosis than someone with two or fewer "yes" answers. Those in the high risk category should immediately discontinue use of or exposure to any drying agents, such as the sun, deodorants, blow dryers, and kitty litter.

IS THERE A SKELETON IN YOUR CLOSET?

By filling out this short survey and sending us your response, you might be the winner of a set of weights, or you might just be out the postage.

Please circle the number next to your response. Thank you for taking part, and remember: Don't press too hard on that pencil, or the point might not be the only thing you break!

1. Do you know anyone who has osteoporosis?
   (Circle as many answers as apply)

   1. Yes, all my family members.

   2. Yes, all my friends.

   3. No, but I don't see well.

2. In your opinion, how likely is it that you will develop osteoporosis sometime in the future?
   (one response only)

   1. I have already been diagnosed with osteoporosis, so don't send me the weights.

   2. Very likely, because I never drink the cream on my Irish Coffee.

   3. Not too likely, because I had a DNA transplant recently.

3. Has a dressmaker ever suggested that you have a bone-density test, or threatened to stop making alterations?

   1. Yes

   2. No

4. Did you know that bone-density tests are available to check for osteoporosis?

   1. I heard about it at the butcher shop.

   2. I thought it was an IQ test.

   3. I have heard of it, but I thought it was a dental procedure.

MIGRAINE
The Ultimate Brainstorm

In spite of intensive medical research, it is still not known why some women are subject to migraine attacks or what triggers them, but current opinion points a guilty finger at computer screens and that special mocha cappuccino you're now addicted to.

Migraines approach with an intensive grip, invading one side of the head and then they begin to throb across the rest of your head like a marching band with an overzealous percussion section. Suddenly, your entire head is aching, the dimmest light seems like 200 watts of unbearable brightness, and you feel that at any moment your lunch may return in an unwelcome form.

Since so many disorders include headaches as a possible symptom, doctors are reluctant to say that migraines are a result of pausin'. However, experience has taught any woman who suffers from hormonal headaches to keep the

Fiorinal next to the Tampax. What the doctor may not tell you is that avoiding certain "triggers" can diminish your chances of incurring the ultimate brainstorm.

Birth control pills: Yes, these can bring on migraines. However, for many women, hot flashes and maternity clothes are less attractive alternatives.

Caffeine: Try to avoid this at all costs. Instead of colas and coffee, think about substituting peppermint tea, meditation, and diesel fuel.

Sugar: It is unfortunate, but the sugary cereal you ate for breakfast could easily turn into Cap'n Crunch's worst nightmare by lunchtime. You can enjoy a wholesome, sugar-free breakfast by whipping up a batch of fibrous bran muffins, popping open a box of unsweetened shredded wheat, or simply foraging in your front yard.

Fumes: Put away the hot glue gun, screw the cap on the paint thinner, and give that nail polish remover to the needy. Exposure to intense fumes can make your blood vessels constrict faster than Martha Stewart can say, "And now let's spray-paint those pinecones."

Pressure: Recent studies have shown that wearing high heels, pantyhose, and business suits can create inordinate pressure on the brain, resulting in excruciating head pain. Consequently, the medical community is now encouraging women in the workplace to impress upon their female colleagues the importance of wearing mumus and flip-flops to work as often as possible.

LOST LIBIDO

Unfortunately, many women experience a loss of passion and accept its demise as a natural part of pausin'. Loss of libido is not cause to sound the alarm, because statistics show that loss of memory, hair, and keys presents far greater problems.

LOST AND FOUND

Don't be foolish enough to think that at this age your sex life will just happen. Reviving a lazy libido is no easy task, so be prepared for some hard work and creative strategies. Check the sizzling tips below to get you back in the sack.

1) *Steamy novels* read late at night, when the kids are asleep, can be an erotic experience for you and your partner, as long as you don't fall asleep too.

2) *Mirrors* overhead can be visually very stimulating to the imagination. Don't spoil the illusion by putting on your glasses.

3) *Aromatherapy* can be an invigorating and pleasurable experience, unless your partner suffers from allergies.

4) *Erotic videos* can offer easy-to-master step-by-step techniques for seduction. Try to select ones that make no mention of food, especially whipped cream. You don't want the urge to eat overriding the urge to make love.

Living Large

AT THE TIME OF OUR BIRTH, most of us are predisposed to a weight and body type that's harder to break out of than Alcatraz. It's no wonder then, that so many women live their lives on rice cakes, carrot sticks, blue milk, and diet cola, while they unsuccessfully try to achieve their "birth weight."

To make matters worse, celebrated over-50 beauties are constantly reminding their overweight sisters how they have managed to pull their careers off the fat-track. Seductively, they sell us diets, machines, and drugs, but not the names of their special-effects make-up artists.

Today, thanks to leaps in modern science, most of us know that dieting is insanity, because menopausal weight gain is tied directly to hormonal changes and not to Twinkies or brownies. Weight gain is one of the most common complaints of pausin', and is rarely covered by insurance.

It's time to face facts and accept yourself. Revel in your accomplishments and not your shortcomings. Learn to accept that you may not lose that last ten pounds, save any money, or take that French course.

Speaking of the French, why not embrace their attitude: "*Mon cherie*, it is better to look like a plum than a prune."

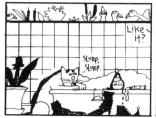 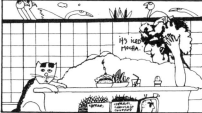

SPREAD SHEET

Don't let the spread sheet alarm you. OK, so some things get bigger while others get smaller, but it's not such a big deal. With just a little maintenance, a lot of patience, and a small fortune, you can look as good as you did on your prom night.

	AGE 20	**AGE 50**
Body Fat	24%	40%
Hair	naturally thick and lustrous	thick and lustrous thanks to: $100 haircut, weekly hot oil treatments, and a commitment to the persistent use of Rogaine
Face	smooth, taut, and glowing	smooth, taut, and glowing thanks to: chemical peels, collagen injections, penetrating deep cleansers, and the ubiquitous mud masque

	AGE 20	AGE 50
Shoulders	straight and strong	the only thing on your body that is getting smaller; it's no problem, however thanks to shoulder pads, which have replaced sanitary pads
Breasts	perky and irresistible	voluptuous and irresistible
Rib Cage & Pelvis	designed for bikinis	designed for babies
Hips & Thighs	underlying bone and muscle structure actually visible at this stage in development	visibly sculpted and well-defined thanks to aerobics, step classes, yoga, push ups, leg lifts, crunches, and lunges
Butt	high, firm, and smooth as a peach	a riper, bigger peach

HOW CAN I TELL IF I'M THE RIGHT WEIGHT?

The good news is, slightly heavier women fare better during menopause.

The ability to "grab a slab" instead of "pinch an inch" is one of the first signs that you've gained enough weight. Other obvious clues are digital scale warnings such as "One at a time, please" or "To be continued."

IS BEING UNDERWEIGHT DANGEROUS?

Statistics compiled by insurance companies, health organizations, and the fashion industry indicate that being underweight is associated with increases in illness and untimely death, but worse than that, your underwear won't stay up.

WHAT CAN I DO TO GAIN WEIGHT?

Try to choose foods from the four main food groups: chips, chocolate, Cokes, and calcium.

RISK MANAGEMENT

Eve craved the apple, hence, all women after her have cravings. Rather than deny yourself, why not just go ahead and indulge, using the Food Cravings Guide Pyramid to help you make intelligent decisions that will minimize the damage? Be sure to eat from the bottom up.

The "Filling Up On Bread Group"

donuts
foccacia
croissants
Belgium waffles
hoagies • garlic
bread • French toast
dumplings • pound
cake • bread pudding
rice pudding • bagels
Pepperridge Farm stuffing
fettucine alfredo • shortbread
Marshmallow Rice Crispie
treats • four-cheese pizza
cinnamon rolls • baguettes

The "Do These Count As Vegetables?" Group

french fries • carrot cake • any
vegetable au gratin • creamed spinach
potato salad • mashed potatoes and gravy
candied yams • onion rings

The "Fruit Flavored" Group

fruit pies • apple cobbler • fruit cake
apple turnovers • caramel apples • banana
splits • pineapple upside-down cake
fruit-flavored Starbursts • strawberry shortcake

The "Very Dairy" Group

cheese doodles • milk shakes • grilled cheese • whipped
cream • Milk Duds • Milky Ways • cream cheese • sundaes

The "High-Fat Protein" Group

bologna • Spam • cashews • sausage balls • organ meats
fried chicken • fast-food burgers • pecan pie • peanut brittle
fish and chips • egg nog • hot dogs • eggs benedict • salami

The "Sweets and Crisps" Group — Use Liberally

M&M's • potato chips • Godiva chocolates • peanut butter fudge
movie popcorn • chocolate mousse • refrigerator cookie dough • jelly
rolls • tollhouse cookies • truffles • Kit-Kat bars • Tootsie Rolls • Pez
Lifesavers • licorice • soft ice cream • oreos • Italian ices • biscotti

THE COMING-OF-AGE CHECKLIST

For most women today, the real reward of pausin' is simply knowing that "health," and not "weight," is the ultimate aphrodisiac of life. Forge ahead, be positive and remember to recite daily the menopause mantra: "Love your love handles."

Check the list below and get acquainted with the new trends in mind and body images for the woman of today. It's OK to eat while you read the list.

Coolish	Foolish
Weighing priorities	Weighing food
Tucking in your children	Tucking your tummy
Crash course on nutrition	Crash diets
Exercising	Victimizing
Cookbooks	Diet books
Skipping rope	Skipping breakfast
Love of food	Fear of fat
High hopes	Tight ropes
Power sit-ups	Liposuction incisions
Rounded hips	Wafer-thin waifs
Eating balanced meals	Ordering "just" an appetizer
Volunteer work	Diet centers
Full bosoms	Wonder bras
Eating out	Eating in the closet

Male Corner

THE PHENOMENON OF PAUSIN' leaves most men bewildered and confused, often questioning the validity of it all. But, hey, guys, unless you keep trading in for newer and younger models, it is not unreasonable to think that you will at one time or another be challenged by a relationship with a woman who happens to be pausin'.

MALE TALES

"I grew my hair and started wearing a ponytail. It threw her into an uncontrollable rage and she shaved her head." —Marc, RCA Record Exec

"I know I'm good in bed, but the crying after sex is really beginning to give me the creeps."
—Tom, photographer

"I always wondered why my parents had twin beds. Now with hot flashes striking, I wish I could get up the courage to ask my wife if it would be OK."
—Michael, commodities trader

"Who would have thought I'd be driving a Lincoln Town Car at my age? But then again, who would have thought that our old Jeep would be hazardous to my wife's bones?" —Al, restaurant owner

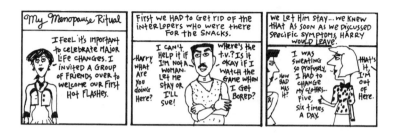

"Even the Stairmaster knew she was lying about her age." —Phil, male dancer

"During our years of marriage, it was the only time I ever complained about running out of toilet paper, and then she went and overcooked my steak on purpose just to be mean." —John, Supreme Court justice

"All I said was 'what happened to the car?' I mean, I didn't accuse her or anything, and bam—suddenly she veered and ran over my foot."
—Ron, real estate developer

TRY A LITTLE TENDERNESS

OK, so there will be nights in January when you feel like one giant goosebump because she has chucked the covers and opened the windows, but try to be empathetic. Of course, you will never really be able to understand what she is going through, any more than she can understand your exasperation after a bad round of golf.

As you begin to see your companion's predictability evaporate, as she struggles to maintain her hormonal harmony, try not to complain. Rather, check out the courses listed below, offered at YMCAs and Elk's lodges across the nation.

• You Can Do Housework Too!
• PMS to Pausin'—Learning When to
  Keep Your Mouth Shut
• How to Fill an Ice Cube Tray
• Reasons to Give Flowers
• You Can Fall Asleep Without It—If You Really Try
• Romanticism—Other Ideas Besides Sex

Past Pause
Milestones In Hormones

HERE WE RESURRECT PAUSE GODDESSES of the past
and honor those of the present.

5000 BC — HOT FLASHES
STONE AGE

*"Once I started taking hormones, I still had hot
flashes, but riding in an open car cooled me off, and
I even learned to stop the car with my feet."*
—Wilma Flintstone

1000 BC — DEPRESSION
MYTHOLOGICAL MOMENTS

*"They say I was responsible for all the trouble that
came out of the box, but Athena, Aphrodite and I had
all become anxious and depressed, and we thought we
would find relief. Now the only thing left is hope."*
—Pandora

1380 BC — DRY SKIN
EGYPTIAN ERA

*"All the oil in my empire won't be able to keep
my skin beautiful once I start pausin'. I'd rather end
it all and be embalmed in my prime."*
—Nefertiti

850 BC — FORGETFULNESS
HEROIC AGE

"While Odysseus was yachting around the Mediterranean slaying beasts and entertaining the sirens, I was stuck at home trying to keep things together. By the time he got back, I'd forgotten who he was but was thankful to have someone around to help watch the sheep."

—Penelope

450 BC — POLITICAL POWER
GREEK EMPIRE

"Although we weren't all as beautiful as Helen, the fact that we all suffered from insomnia gave us plenty of time to think of our plan to stop the war."

—The Trojan Women

500 AD — HOT FLASHES
DARK AGES

*"In the days of old,
when knights were bold,
Pausin' was difficult
(if you lived that long).
But drafty castles
and a dip in the moat
cooled down my hot flashes
without a doubt!"*

—Guinevere

1380 AD — POST-MENOPAUSAL ZEST
THE MIDDLE AGES

"Pausin' on the pilgrimage was not easy for a woman my age, but by staying out of the pubs, I kept a straight head and always got what I wanted— the friar, the knight, and young student alike."
—Wife of Bath

1500 AD — TRANQUILITY
THE RENAISSANCE

"A good glass of Italian wine can produce a mysterious smile on any woman plagued by pausin'."
—Mona Lisa

1776 AD — FORGETFULNESS
REVOLUTIONARY ERA

"I thought I would never get that flag finished on time. Every time I got up to get a snack or walk to the outhouse, I lost my needle or misplaced my glasses. I had to do it over twice to get the number of stars right."
—Betsy Ross

1820 AD — WEIGHT
THE NAPOLEONIC PERIOD

"When I started pausin', my body changed. The styles of the period allowed more room in the hips and waist. Coincidentally, I could breathe again."
—Josephine Bonaparte

1880 AD — MIGRAINES
VICTORIAN AGE

"Taking care of the wounded soldiers was nothing compared to nursing the crabby gals who complained of migraines."

—Florence Nightingale

1930 AD — HOT FLASHES
THE NEW DEAL

"When I had hot flashes, I would feel free to remove my tweeds and undies, but I never considered taking off my pearls or gloves."

—Eleanor Roosevelt

1950 AD — OSTEOPOROSIS
THE COMIC STRIP ERA

"If I had known about shark cartilage in my day, I would have had the strength to kick Popeye's butt."

—Olive Oyl

2000 AD — HOT FLASHES
THE NEW MILLENNIUM

"Can I get any hotter?" —Madonna

Future Pause
2001: A Hormone Odyssey

WELCOME TO PLANET PAUSE, the hottest place in cyberspace. Since the future is not what it used to be, you can now journey across your computer screen and explore pausin' styles from Budapest to Bora Bora, without ever leaving your couch and chips.

Never mind that you can't program a VCR, much less a computer. Consider the Hormone Superhighway, the interactive forum where women will compare prescription prices, share experiences, and lend support.

While you are spacing out on Planet Pause, stop at the planetarium to find out how the movements and positions of the heavenly bodies control and influence your behavior.

SURFING THE HORMONE SUPERHIGHWAY

Check out these real internet websites with information on menopause:

FEMINA
http://www.femina.com
A vast search engine of various women's sites

HEALTH AND SCIENCE WEB PAGE
http://www.health-science.com/
Features the Natural Progesterone and Women's Health Page (www.health-science.com/health/htm), which includes "A Guide to Understanding and Controlling PMS, Fertility, Menopause, and Osteoporosis." Contains: "what doctors don't tell you about menopause."

POWER SURGE
http://members.aol.com/dearest/index.html
"Online Resource for Menopausally Savvy Women."
Also features online chats, AOL's Women's Interest Channel, Community Conference Online, regularly-scheduled physicians (chat), recent chat guests include Gail Sheehy, Lonnie Barbach, and Letty Cottin Pogrebin. Also weekly talks with naturopaths, authors and doctors.

THE MENOPAUSE LINK
http://www.progest.com
Features "Take Control of Your Health," health resources, chats with doctors, Pro-Gest page, and a page of menopausal experiences. Sponsored by Transitions for Health.

A FRIEND INDEED
http://www.odyssee.net/~janine
A menopausal newsletter edited by Janine O'Leary Cobb.
Has United States and Canadian resources, and back issues
of the newsletter.

MENOPAUSE
http://www.yahoo.com/Health/Women_s_Health/menopause/
Menopausal resources from Yahoo's contents.

WOMEN'S HEALTH INTERACTIVE
http://www.womens-health.com
Has menopause/HRT section (www.womens-health.
com/rcs_ml.html). Their Health and Science section also
has information on understanding and controlling
menopausal symptoms and hormonal changes.

A VIRTUAL WOMEN'S CLINIC FOR WOMEN IN THEIR SECOND FORTY YEARS
http://www.womencare.com
Headed by Karen Lee, RN.

HYSTERIA PUBLICATIONS' WEB PAGE
http://www.hysteriabooks.com
Visit our web page to link to all these sites.

THE ESTROLOGICAL CHART

While cruising the Internet may not appeal to all women, controlling one's destiny does. Here's a chart that can help you guide your pause. Take advantage of all the hidden powers of your sign and check out the planetary alignment for your month of birth. See what messages it holds for you.

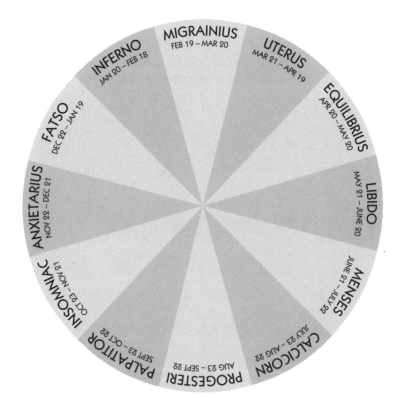

THE HORMONOSCOPE

Libido: Women born under this sign will experience a drastic drop in their response to passion during pausin'. Venus will intercept only rarely; temporarily, desire and lust are replaced by apathy and indifference. It is best not to cover up negative feelings during this period; this will only leave your mate feeling hostile and frustrated. Try to be tactful when saying "no," and rest assured that a good shopping spree can replace any pleasures that you might be missing.

Menses: Turbulence invades your cosmic flow and dominates your conscious mind. Harmony can be brought about only when Menses aligns with Mars. Unfortunately, this union will take place less and less frequently as time marches on, so learn to go with the flow.

Calcicorn: Symbolizes strength and urges you to straighten up. Calcicorn rules the hips and wrists, and warns you that your future happiness depends on how you channel the cosmic flow of milk. This is a period of endings and beginnings, so remember that your losses can always be replaced by something better (like a new plastic hip).

Progesteri: The full moon in Progesteri marks a major transition for women. Linked with serious losses, lunar aspects indicate tension with medical advisors, loved ones and colleagues. Only when Progesteri enters Uterus that can you expect to achieve harmony on the homefront.

Palpitator: Listen to your heart. This sign once guided your love life with reckless abandon, but now these palpitations and irregular thumps are signs of fatigue and exhaustion brought on by pausin'. Most women have difficulty recognizing that the pulsations that once drove them wild now need to be tamed with Chinese medicines and herbal teas. Remember, an affair is not a good idea at this time in your life and could potentially endanger your health.

Insomniac: Needless to say, women born under this sign will be heavily influenced by the moon and Jay Leno during their pausin' years. With many planets retrograde during the night, your restless nature surfaces, compromising your daily life to a significant degree. Insomniacs are often fired from their jobs for repeatedly showing up late or for absences caused by falling asleep after lunch. Use time in the evening to get in touch with your soul and that strange creature that has moved into your body. Or, better yet, get rid of the fuzzy things in the back of your refrigerator.

Anxietarius: Slow the pace and take more time for inner voyages. Since Anxietarius is not compatible with other planets, those under this sign are fated with a case of frazzled nerves. Poor decisions such as making three commitments for the same evening, or promising to help a friend move next weekend while forgetting your daughter's graduation, are triggered by the opposition of planets circling the path of Anxietarius. Anxietarians are also accident-prone, with frequent trips to therapists increasing the possibility of injury.

Fatso: The influence of Pluto and the Pillsbury doughboy could cause you to put on a few extra pounds. Make light of earthly concerns and consider this a time of growth and expansion.

Inferno: If you are born under this sign, you can expect things to heat up during pause, because Infernos like to align with Mercury (the fire sign) which brings on hot flashes so intense that the blaze can be extinguished only by the intercession of a water sign. The more well-heeled pauser will want to take comfort at the nearest spa or exotic resort, but for the rest of us, the nearest fire hydrant will achieve the same result.

Migranius: When several planets meet up and clash, Migranius goes to work trying to regain her position in the hormonal orbit. Sadly, this shifting of the powers destines many women to experience throbbing, pounding, relentless health challenges. Communication is the cornerstone for all progress, so be sure to give fair warning to those around you when you feel this collision approaching and avoid all coffee bars.

Uterus: Be prepared for upheaval. You must learn to avoid sentimentality and nostalgia, because this may be the time to say goodbye to those things that have outlived their purpose.

Equilibrius: Women bearing this sign must strive to maintain balance and resist the temptation to abuse medication and loved ones no matter how bad things get. This is a critical time during which constant supervision is required. You may have to take an unplanned trip because a change of scenery is just what your family asked the doctor to order.

Pause & Reflect

NOW THAT YOU HAVE READ *THE NOISY PASSAGE*, you have reached a new hormonally incorrect understanding of life that will help you meet all your "uter-lateral" challenges with pills, patches, and humor. To reflect on what you have just read or simply to refresh your memory, take this simple test designed to measure your current hormonal comprehension, as well as your reading ability. Above all, don't be upset if you don't do well the first time (memory loss is usually temporary). You can take the test over and over again until you achieve a satisfactory score. Pick up a #2 pencil. Let's begin.

1. Estrogen and progesterone are . . .
   (a) Approved by the Surgeon General to dispense in public schools
   (b) Magicians
   (c) The names of Jane Fonda's children

2. Hot flashes are signals that . . .
   (a) Rain is in the forecast
   (b) You ate too much Indian food
   (c) Your car has broken down

3. Provera is . . .
   (a) The part of speech that modifies a verb
   (b) A province in France
   (c) Given to pilots to make them more alert

4. Some minor drawbacks of Hormone

Replacement Therapy are . . .
(a) Sudden career changes
(b) Simultaneous weight gain, insomnia, memory loss, incontinence and stubble
(c) Frizzy hair (on the chin and chest)

5. Vaginal jellies are . . .
(a) Low in fat
(b) Worn mostly at the beach
(c) Ordered from Harry and David's Catalogue

6. Menopause begins when . . .
(a) Your credit card is declined
(b) You swear off men
(c) You are bored
(d) Your Rolodex becomes a blunt instrument

7. Unusual vaginal bleeding is a sign of . . .
(a) Bad hair coloring
(b) Pants that are too tight
(c) Religious superiority
(d) Acupuncture abuse

8. Calcium is . . .
(a) A new fragrance by Calvin Klein
(b) The capital of India
(c) Intended to be freebased
(d) A condiment

9. Middle-age spread is best described as . . .
(a) The time in history when knights were bold
(b) More affordable than butter
(c) A ladies' luncheon

10. Estrogen patches are . . .
    (a) Easy to sew on jackets
    (b) The best way to stop smoking
    (c) The preferred eyewear of pirates

11. Mammograms are . . .
    (a) Mother's Day greetings
    (b) A small unit of measure
    (c) Used to make crust for cheesecake

12. Female gynecologists are more honest than . . .
    (a) Auto mechanics
    (b) Clergymen
    (c) The President
    (d) The First Lady

13. Male gynecologists are really . . .
    (a) Gem specialists looking for diamonds
        in the rough
    (b) Frustrated spelunkers

14. Calcium implant procedures are usually
    performed . . .
    (a) At Carnegie Hall
    (b) By dental hygenists
    (c) After approval from the co-op board
    (d) To prevent a cheesecake deficit
    (e) After foreplay

15. More than 7 million women rely on premarin to . . .
    (a) Sweeten their morning coffee
    (b) Put their children to bed at night
    (c) Get their dishes clean

16. Breast self-exams are . . .
    (a) Ordered by mail
    (b) Good because you can't be caught cheating
    (c) Banned by the Catholic Church

17. Anxiety can best be described as . . .
    (a) A song played at New Year's Eve parties
    (b) DNA by-product
    (c) Number one killer of women
    (d) One panty liner plus five cups of herbal tea plus one three-hour movie

18. Menstruation is . . .
    (a) A thick, hearty Italian soup
    (b) The mark at the end of a sentence
    (c) A hex placed on you by the sanitary napkin conglomerate when you were thirteen

19. PMS is . . .
    (a) An ingredient to keep food fresh
    (b) A maneuver taught in driver's ed
    (c) A pesticide banned in the 1950s
    (d) The monogram on Paul Simon's luggage

Glossary

BLADDER—(blad-err) n.
To flow on endlessly about nothing or to leak out secret information.

BLADDER CONTROL—(blad-err con-troll) n.
More strategic than arms control.

BONE DENSITY—(bone den-city) n.
Stupidity regarding the female skeleton.

BLOAT—(blow-ta) v.
To become a flotation device.

CALCIUM—(cal-see-yum) n.
Determining your future physique through a mathematical process.

CHANGE OF LIFE—(chain-ja life) n.
Process not as smelly as change of diaper.

CELLULITE—(cell-u-lite) n.
The low-fat variety of a cell.

ENERGY LOSS—(in-er-gee los) n.
Blackout from six-way conference calling or childcare.

EXERCISE—(x-or-size) v.
Either you do, or you don't.

ESTROGEN—(astro-gen) n.
Take it or leave it!

ESTRACE CREAM—(s-trace creem) n.
A cream that erases vaginal wrinkles.

FLUID RETENTION—(flu-id-re-ten-shun) n.
When your waist and ankles are the same size.

FERTILE—(fur-til) n.
What you (and your imagination) were before you got married.

FATIGUE—(fat-eeg) n.
A uniform worn by middle-aged women to camouflage the impact of pausin'.

GYNECOLOGIST—(guy-neck-col-o-gist) n.
The guy who knows you inside out.

HEAVY PERIODS—(heh-vee pee-ree-uds) n.
See Rubens or Flemish art of 1600.

HEADACHE—(head-ayke) n.
Like heartache, but up higher.

HORMONES—(her-moans) n.
The groaning sounds made by a pausin' woman.

HOT FLASH—(hot-flash) n.
The latest fashion bulletin.

HYSTERECTOMY—(his-tor-wrecked-tummy) n.
History of the anatomy.

H.R.T.—(H-R-T) n.
English acronym for Her Royal Temper, a term referring to the Queen's mood swings.

INSOMNIA—(in-some-knee-a) n.
An all nighter.

INCONTINENCE—(in-con-tin-ents) n.
Garden Club excursions between the United States and Canada.

IRRITABILITY—(ear-it-ability) n.
A violent trait shared by pausin' women and pitbulls.

IRREGULAR PERIODS—(ir-reg-u-lar pee-ree-uds) n.
The use of erratic punctuation.

KEGEL—(kay-gul) n.
Low-calorie substitute for a bagel.

LIBIDO—(lib-bee-doe) n.
Essential attribute for becoming a U.S. Senator.

MENOPAUSE—(man-o-paws) n.
Footprints of prehistoric man.

MIGRAINE—(my-grain) n.
Tasty hormone-frosted cereal recommended by most doctors.

MEMORY LOSS—(mem-or-ee los) n.
Easier to replace than hair loss: see benefits of mental floss.

MOOD SWINGS—(mood-swings) n.
Gym apparatus designed for people on Prozac.

NIGHT SWEATS—(nite-swets) n.
Brightly colored day-glo jogging attire.

N.D.E.—(near death experience) n.
Your mother's version of pausin'.

NERVOUSNESS—(ner-vus-nus) n.
Becoming agitated or unsteady when receiving
your balance from ATM machine;
see: Declined credit.

OVULATION—(ov-u-lay-shun) n.
Game of chance similar to Concentration, where
the winner ends up with the most eggs.

PALPITATION—(pal-pit-a-shun)
A beat hard to dance to.

P.M.S.—(pee-m-s) n.
Makes you C:R.Y.

PROVERA— (pro-vera) n.
A tropical plant used to treat third-degree hot flash burns.

PROGESTERONE—(pro-gest-er-own) n.
A partner of Estrogen who might think nothing of
leaving you high and dry.

PREMARIN—(pre-mar-in) n.
Fruit-flavored, chewable vitamins.

PELVIS—(pel-vis) n.
The female counterpart to Elvis.

PLASTIC SURGERY—(plaz-tik sur-ger-ee) n.
The craft of making Barbie dolls.

RAGE—(ray-ge) n.
The current craze of pausin'.

STRESS—(stres) n.
The build-up of pressure brought on by comparison shopping.

SKIPPING PERIODS—(skip-ing-pee-ree-ods) n.
Not as aerobic as hopping or stepping, but a good way
to stay fit.

SUPPORT GROUPS—(sup-port-grups) n.
Undergarment manufacturers with the mature
woman in mind.

TESTOSTERONE—(test-ost-er-own) n.
The real last name of Italian Stallion, Sylvester.

UTERUS—(U-ter-us) n.
Slang: "In uterus we trust."

VAGINAL ATROPHY—(va-gi-nul a-tro-fee) n.
A trophy for years of service rendered.

WEIGHT—(wait; rhymes with ate) n.
When you have everything to lose and nothing to gain;
see: one size fits all.

About the authors

MARIE EVANS

Marie-Christine, a true Southern belle, was born sometime in March A.D. Feeling repressed in her native South, she fled North in order to pursue her lifelong dream of becoming a painter. Finally a liberated woman in New York, Marie wasted no time in marrying, thus ending her career as a painter. Two perfect daughters later, Marie, wishing to give thanks for her good fortune, has become a committed advocate for women's issues. You will find this mom behind the wheel of "Powder Puff," her pink, hormone-injected flashmobile, demonstrating Kegel exercises in front of Victoria's Secret on Mondays and Wednesdays. Marie has unselfishly donated her mind and body to science (her body was rejected). Holding both her BFA and MFA degrees, she is currently working toward her PMS degree from the correspondence school of The Convent of Hormonal Sorrows.

ANN SHAKESHAFT

Ann, a fashionable former art director at *Mademoiselle*, *Glamour*, *Seventeen* and *Woman's Day*, now fills her prescriptions and her days color-coding and artistically arranging her wide assortment of pills. At her young age of forty-something, Ann is the envy of both her friends. She is attractive and fit and shows no signs of the midlife crisis which she has undergone. Ann has unexpectedly survived one marriage, two children, a hysterectomy after each child, and numerous renovations on her home (none on her body). Today with the help of the corner clairvoyant, her manicurist, personal trainer, hairdresser (specializing in transplants), six-packs of anti-aging cream, and frequent trips to Canyon Ranch, Ann has become the woman she used to be. Her husband and children visit on weekends.

92 / The Noisy Passage: Baby Boomers Do Menopause

Other great titles from Hysteria Publications:

BOOKS

Getting in Touch with Your Inner Bitch
by Elizabeth Hilts (Paperback, $7.95)
Our best seller. Release that untapped power that
knows what she knows and isn't afraid to say so!

*Dates for the Greats: A Personal Ads Parody
from Adam & Eve to Sigmund Freud*
by Doris Chelmow and Harold Rand (Paperback, $8.95)
Parody personals paired with a veritable rogue's gallery
of historical lovelorns.

A Useless Guide to WindBlows95
by Murkysoft (Paperback, $7.95)
Your computer, your appliances and your life will
never be the same!

Pandemonium: Or, Life with Kids
a collection of parental humor (Paperback, $7.95)
From the "Parental Aptitude Test" to "The Young Adults
Return," Pandemonium is the only parenting book that
takes you all the way.

'Cause I'm the Mommy (That's Why!)
by Donna Black (Paperback, $7.95)
A writing mom laughs at those moments all mothers
go through. With cartoons by Nicole Hollander.

The Noisy Passage
by Marie Evans and Ann Shakeshaft (Paperback, $8.95)
Speed down the Hormone Superhighway with this
fast-paced farce.

CALENDARS

Sylvia's Cosmic Companion:
A Guide to Keeping Your Goddess Happy
A 1997 Astrological Cartoon Engagement Calendar
by Nicole Hollander ($12.95)
It's small enough to carry in your purse!

Sylvia's Cosmic Companion:
Let the Goddess Run Your Life in 1997
An Astrological Cartoon Wall Calendar
by Nicole Hollander ($12.95)
Both formats include an astrological goddess cartoon for
each month, birthdates of secular goddesses, quotations
about the heavens, and goddess asteroid information.

Personally Yours: A Personal Ads
Parody Calendar for 1997
by Doris Chelmow and Harold Rand
(Wall calendar, $12.95)
Parody personal ads plus birthdates of famous and
infamous lovers, quotes about love gone awry and
special days related to romance.

To place an order by Visa or MasterCard,
please call us at (800) 784-5244.

Hysteria Publications is a book and calendar publisher dedicated to humor. We'll gladly consider your manuscript or book proposal. Please send submissions to:

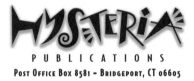

Please include SASE and phone number with all submissions and allow six weeks for a reply.